Budding Brayton

Using two switches for one activity

Created by Luke Thompson

Co-author Caroline Bennett

Illustrated by Kat Willott

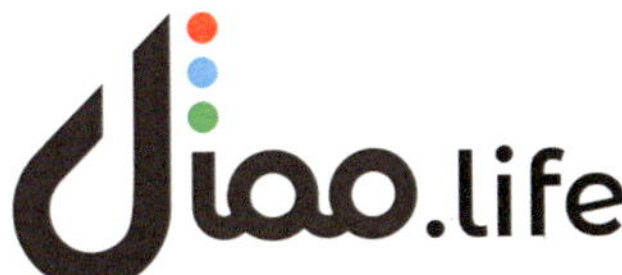

Published by Jiao Ltd
Jiao.life

Scan the QR codes to access the digital book or listen to the audio book.

Audiobook

Digital Book

The Seven Stages of Switch Development

Budding Brayton is part of the Switch Heroes, social stories created to support switch-users with their Switch progression. The Switch Heroes series is part of the Seven Stages of Switch Development, created by Occupational Therapist and AT specialist Luke Thompson.

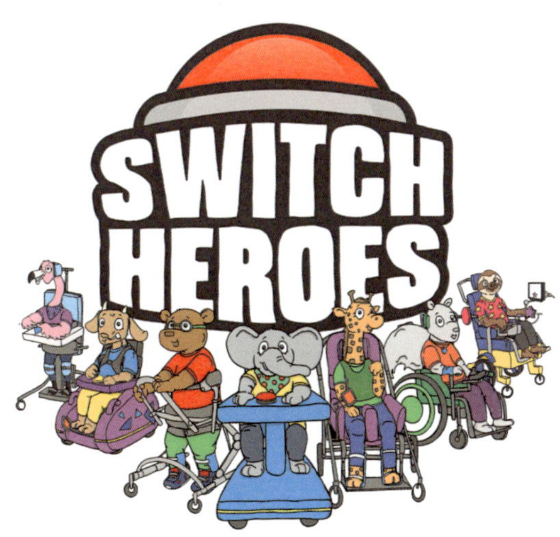

Brayton’s got a big voice

A speaker makes the sound

He gives it just one push

His voice is all around

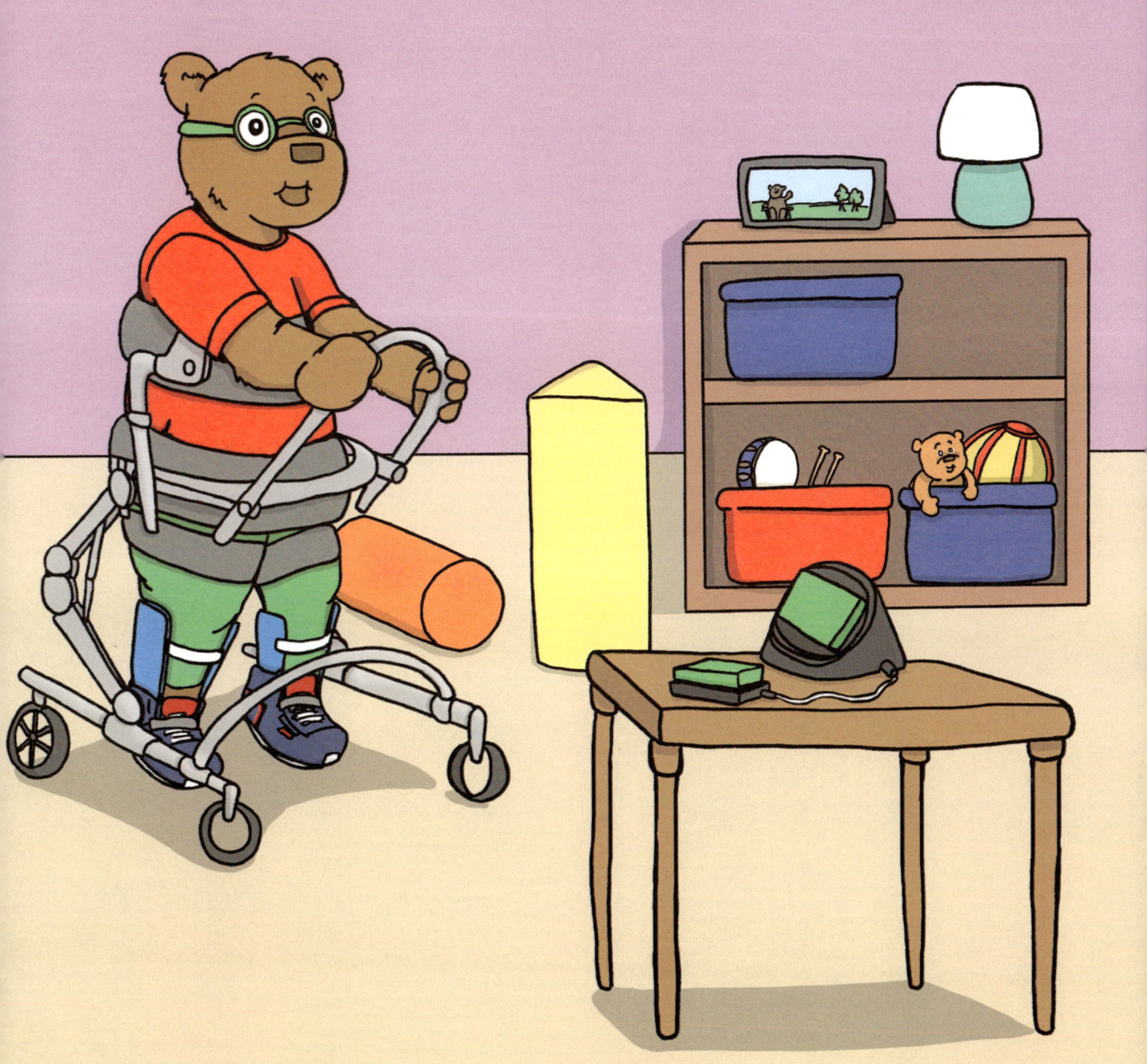

Brayton's got a big voice

His switch helps him say

All of the important things

He really wants to say

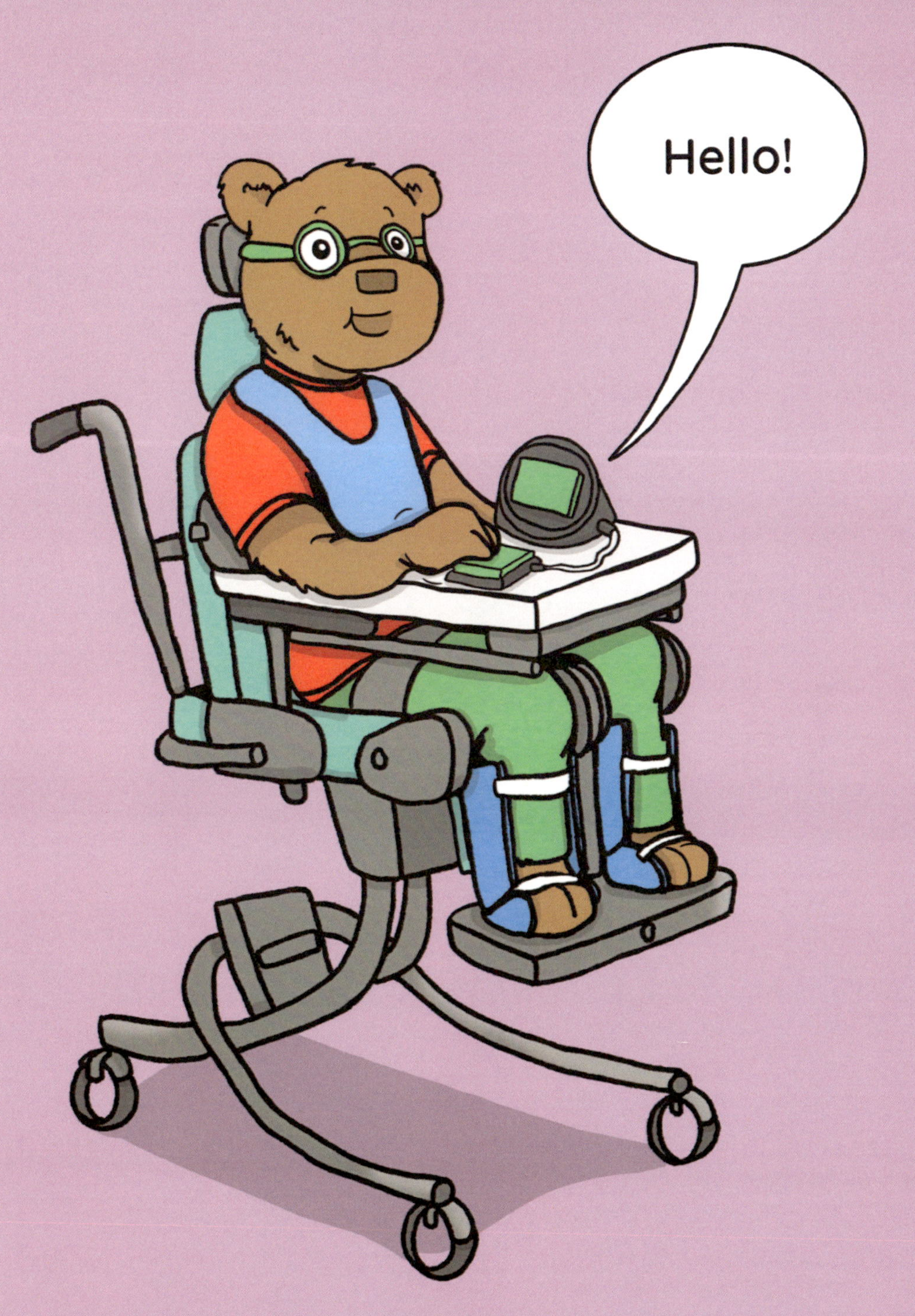
Hello!

Let’s get your two
green rectangles

They make different sounds

One switch asks to,
‘build a tower’

The other, ‘knock it down!’

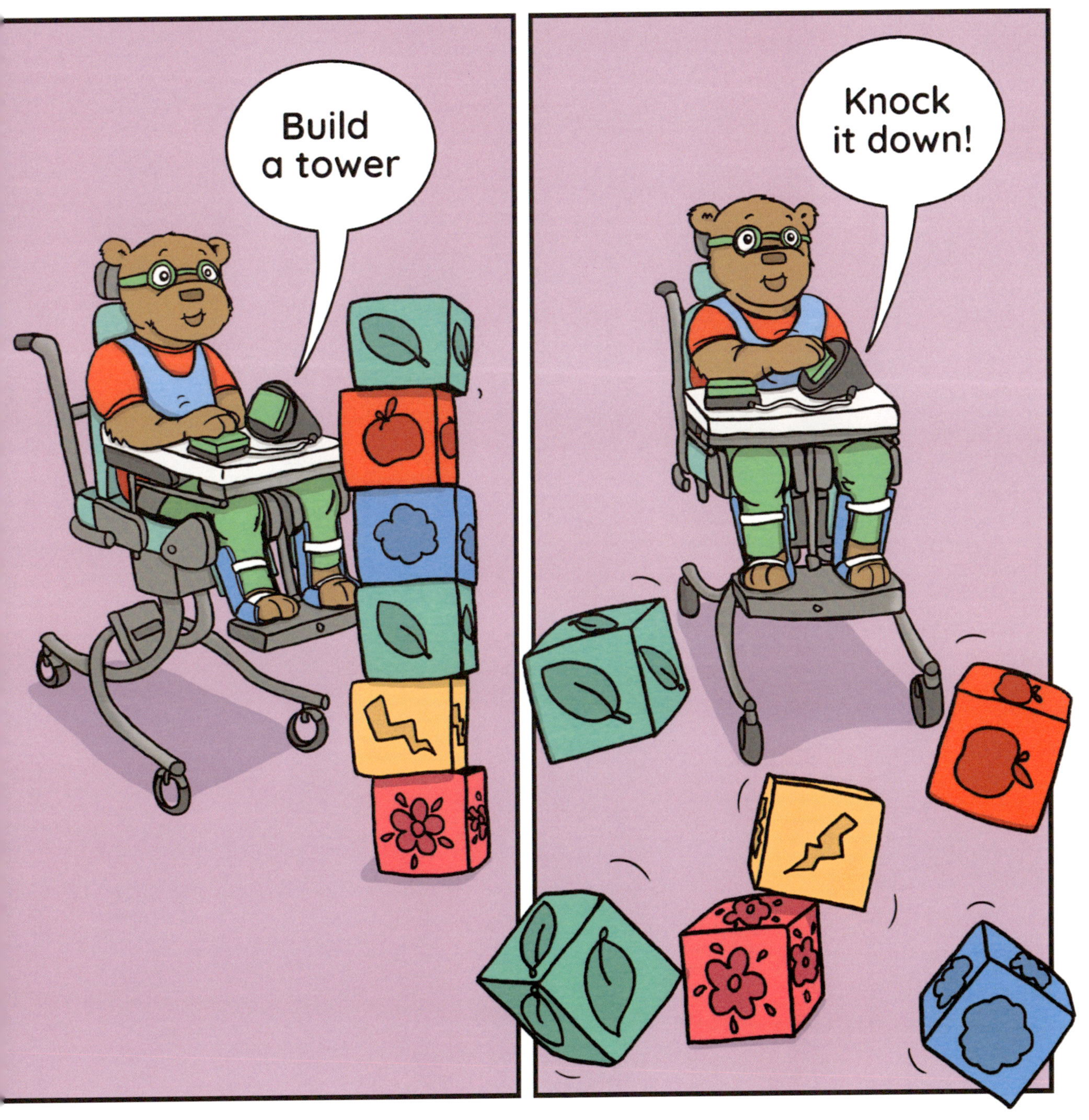
Build
a tower
Knock
it down!

You can use two switches
When you have things to say
You can use two switches
Move your chair each way

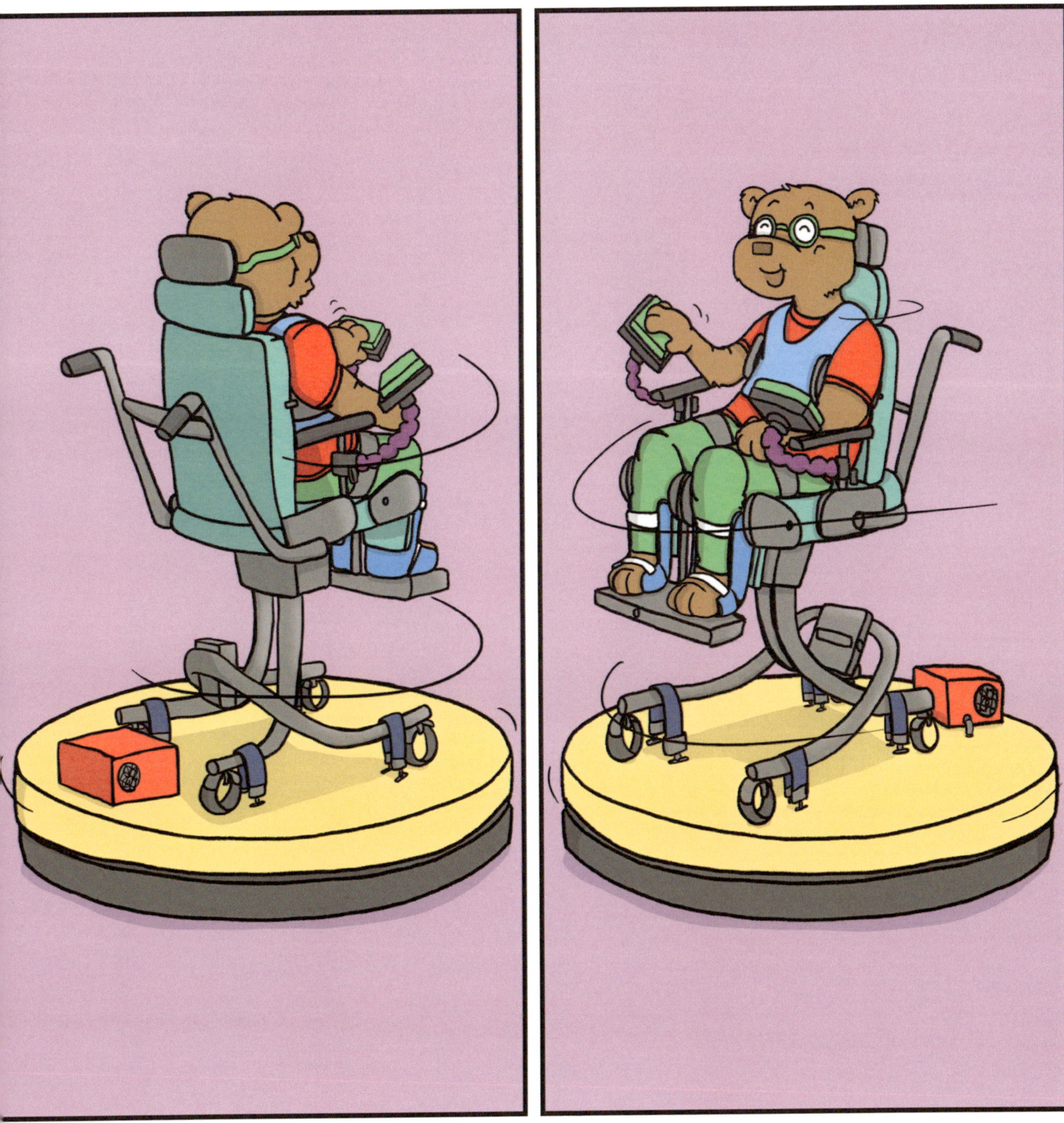

You can use two switches

To play a funny game

Now you’re using switches

Things won’t be the same

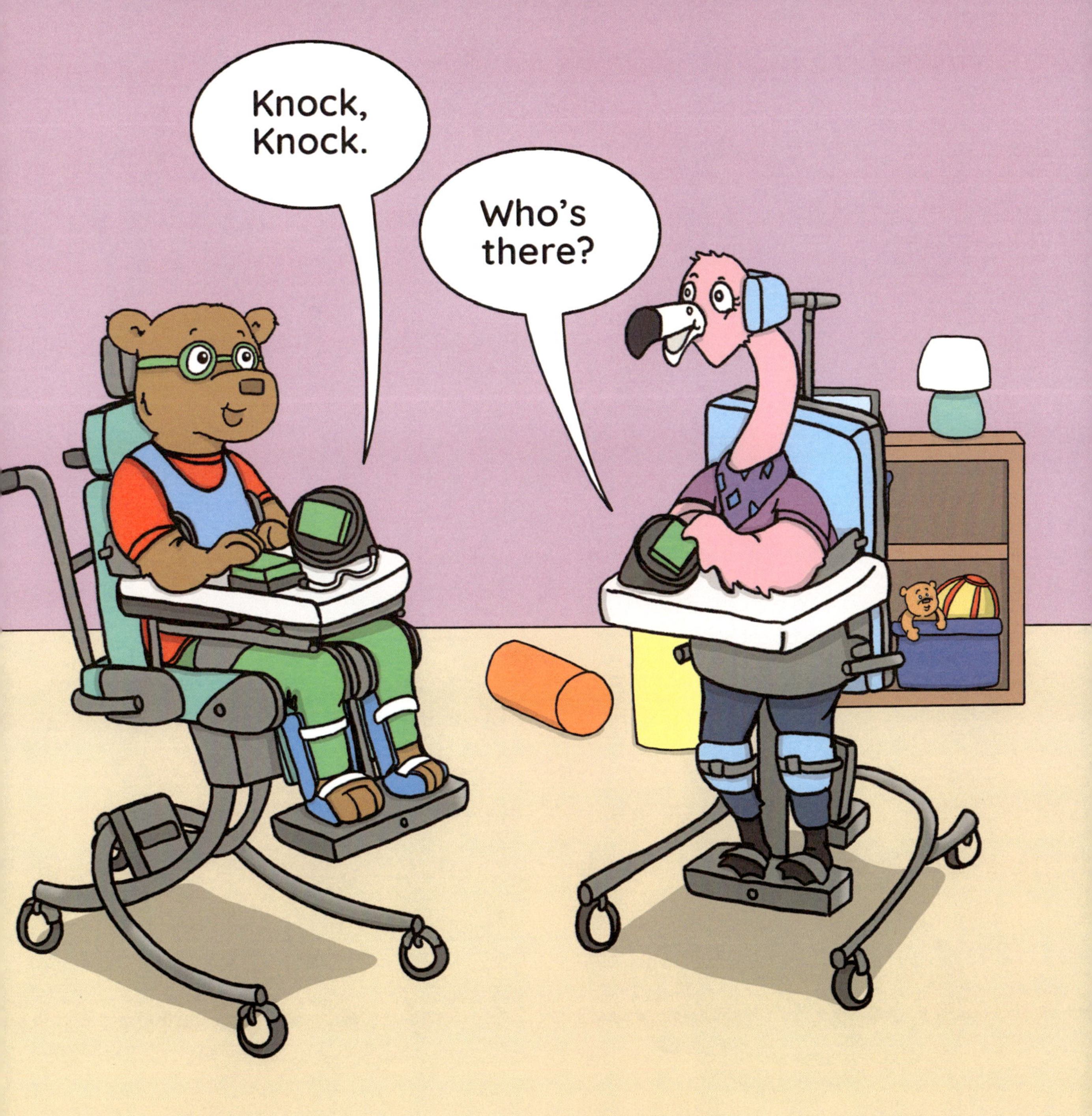
Knock,
Knock.
Who's
there?

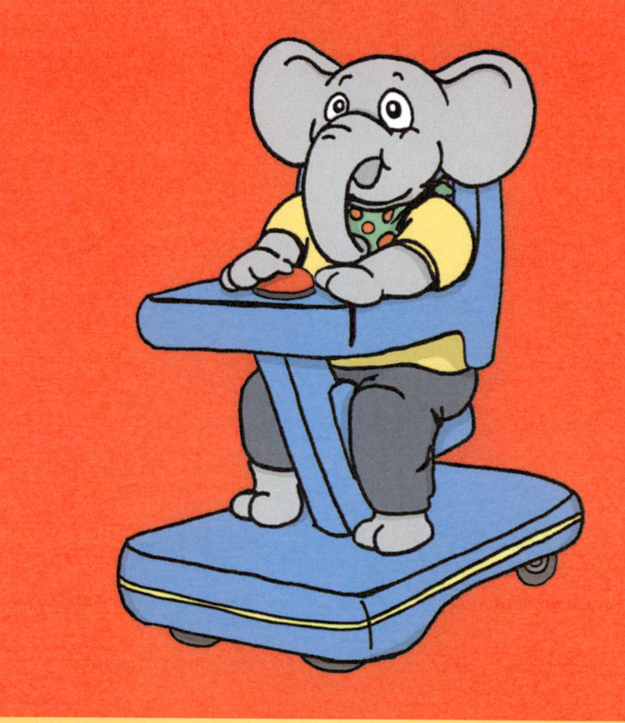
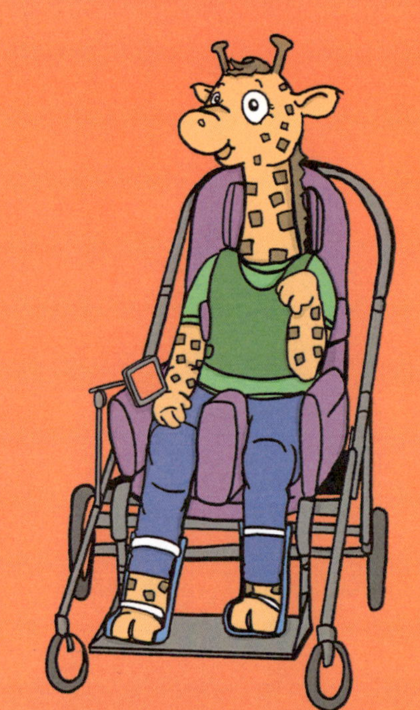
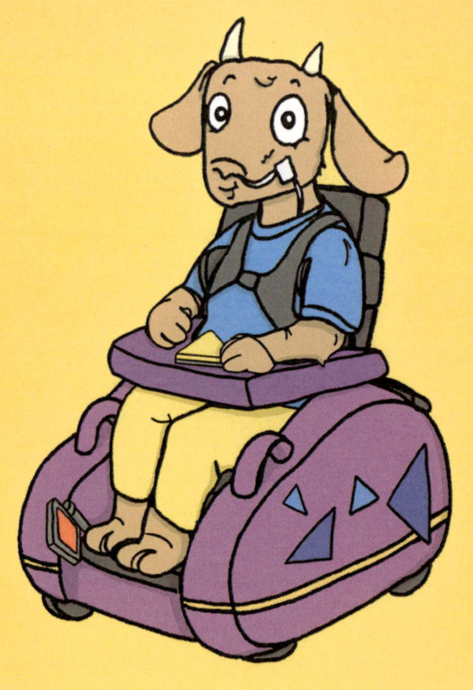
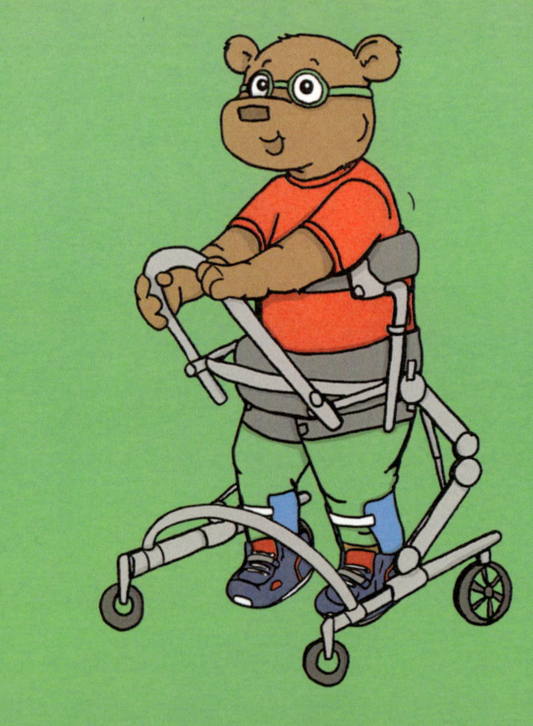

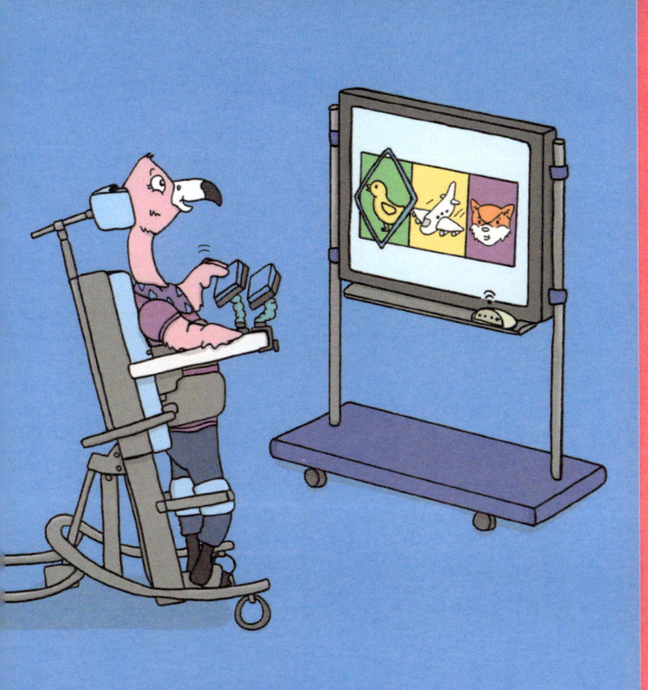

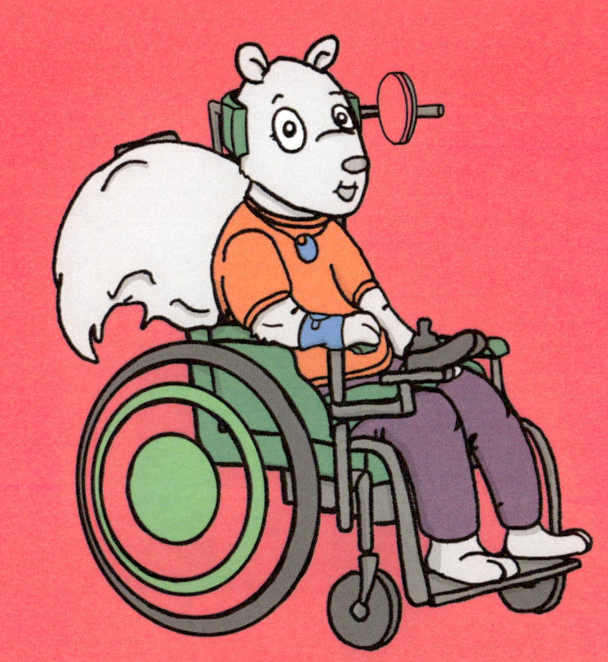

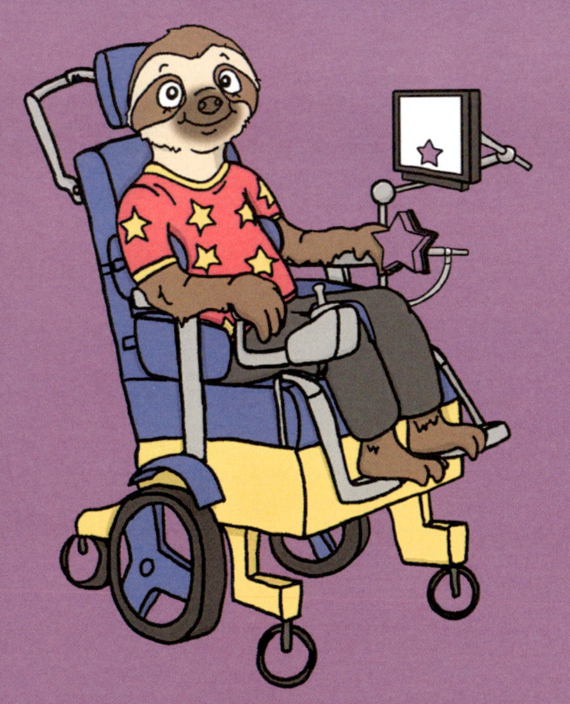

Photo of you!

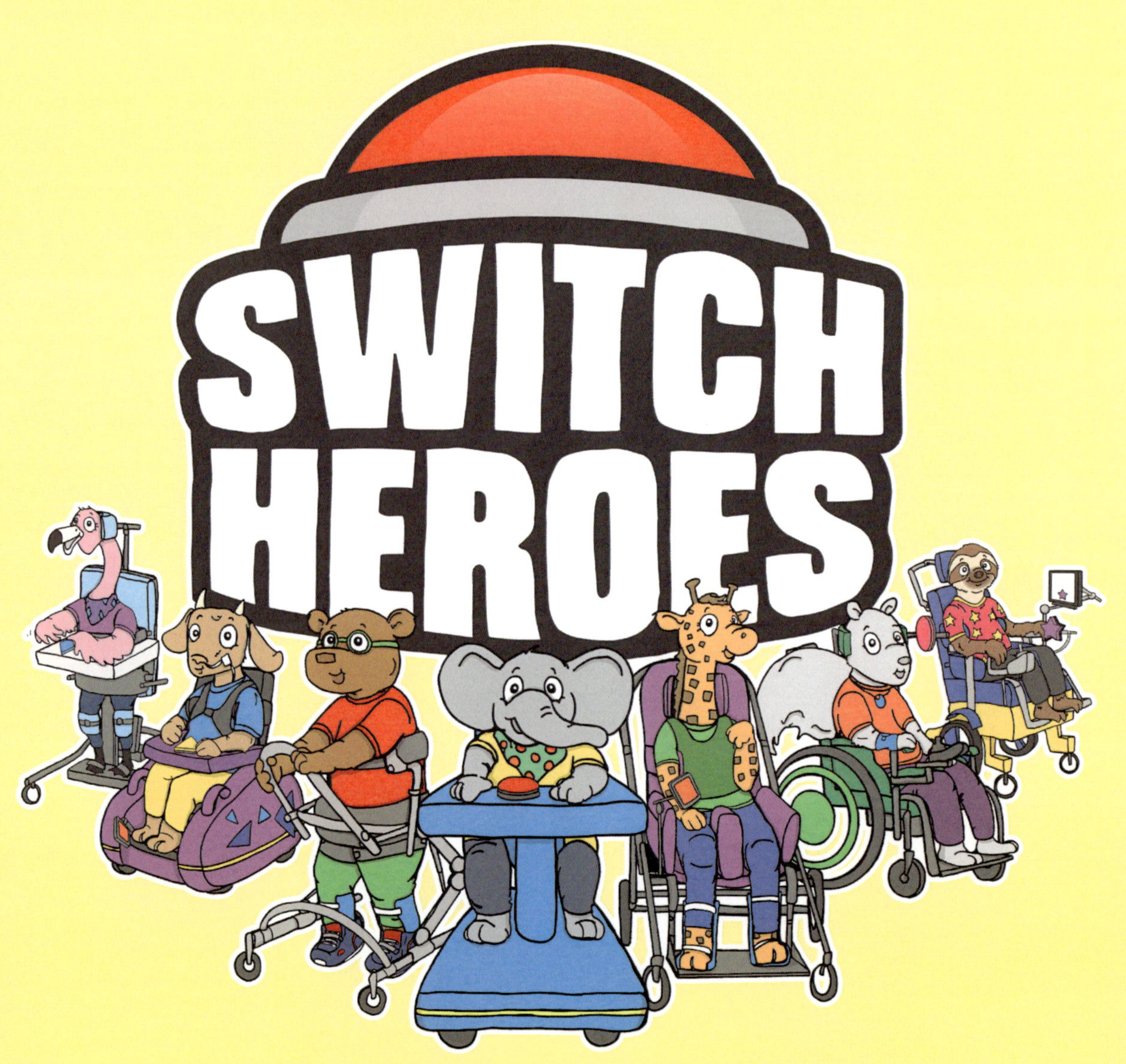
SWITCH HEROES

The Seven Stages of Switch Development

The Seven Stages of Switch Development is a resource designed for switch-users, their families, caregivers and those who assist them in using switches. It features child-friendly characters and stories that support everyones learning.

The framework provides a helpful reference for measuring and tracking progress while offering flexibility to accommodate the unique needs and preferences of each switch-user.

Written directly to the switch-user, the framework can be read to them if they are unable to read it themselves. Our aim is to ensure that those supporting the child/switch-user can prioritise the child's needs and perspective in the process of developing their switch skills. We have seen the impact of involving the child in the learning process. Seeking their input and feedback regularly empowers them to take an active role in their development and combat learned helplessness.

Adapted from: Bean, I. (2011). Switch Progression Learning Journeys Road Map. Inclusive Technology.
Burkhart, L. (2018). Stepping Stones to Switch Access. Perspectives of the ASHA Special Interest Groups, 3(12), pp.33-44. doi:https://doi/10.1044/persp3.sig12.33.

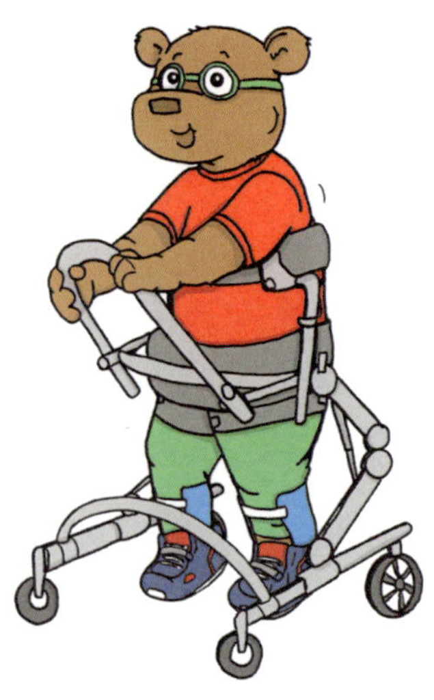

Stage 4
Using two switches for one activity
Budding Brayton the Bear
Rectangle/Green

Definition

Budding Brayton is the stage where you use two switches with different actions for one activity. Let's say you want to build something - you can press one switch to start building, and then press another switch to knock it down. Or, you can use one switch to say, 'go' and another switch to say, 'stop' and play a game with your helpers. There are lots of online games that use two switches that you can start to explore. Make sure you start with simple two-switch games and avoid scan and select activities. Here is a list of types of two-switch computer activities in order of difficulty (easy to hard):

Free choice: Each switch activates an action from choice of two (e.g. a character singing/dancing)

On/off choice: First switch starts an action and the second switch interrupts that action (build, build – knock down OR play music - stop)

Rotate complete: The first switch rotates through options and the second completes (e.g. food options for crocodile - crocodile eats)

Sequential actions: The first switch completes several steps and the second switch either repeats an action and/or completes the activity (builds, builds, stops - launches rocket)

Milestones

- You understand that the two switches connect the two actions to form a sequence for a specific activity
- You can independently select and activate the appropriate switches for the desired action specifically when one switch becomes dormant and the second is required to complete the activity
- You can anticipate, plan and problem solve for the necessary sequence of actions using the two switches – for example when the first switch sequence is complete you will quickly move to the second switch to complete the activity
- You can repeat the activity using the same sequence of switches consistently
- You can generalise the skill to different activities and settings that require the use of two switches
- You have become increasingly proficient at using your body to activate two switches for one activity

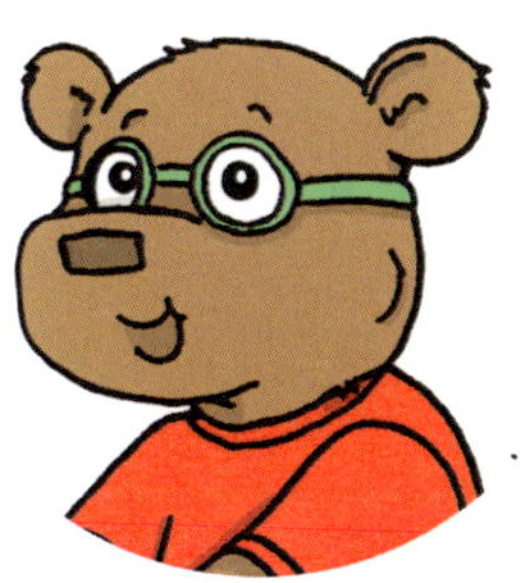

Activities

- Incorporating two different switch toys into one game. For example, one switch activates a toy that moves or dances, while the other plays music. The goal of the game is to have the toy dance whenever the music plays and stop when the music stops. This encourages the child to coordinate both switches and engage with the activity in a fun, interactive way
- Programme two voice-output switches (or one with two-switch options) to give different commands in a fun game (e.g., 'clap your hands' and 'do a star jump')
- Computer games: there are lots of two-switch computer activities. Try simple activities that allow each switch to play a different sound or function. You can progress to more complicated two-switch activities where one switch works first and the second is redundant/plays a repeat action. Then when the steps are complete the first switch becomes redundant and the second switch finishes the activity

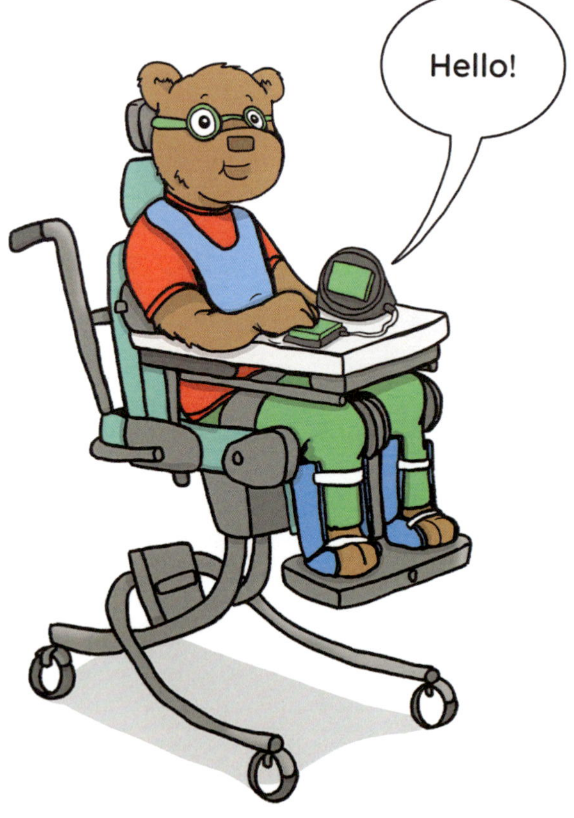

Top tips

- Provide clear and consistent feedback to reinforce successful use of both switches together
- Use activities that require the child to use both switches to achieve a specific outcome
- Review switch positioning and supports with the child, considering whether guides or barriers are necessary to differentiate between switch presses and reduce accidental activations

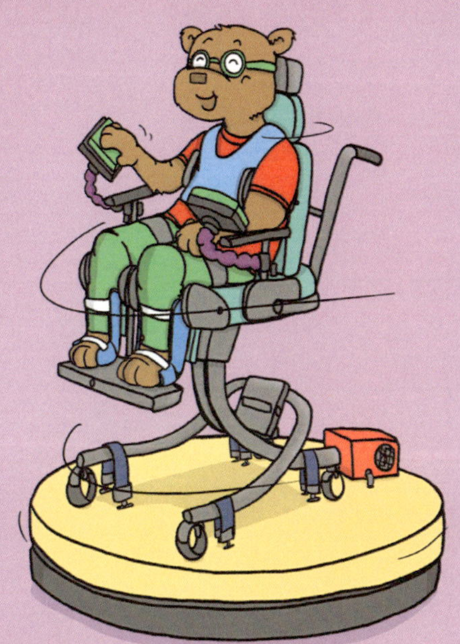

Instead of a prompt hierarchy where the type of prompt increase in support level, we recommend our one prompt switch support cycle. Find out more at Jiao.life

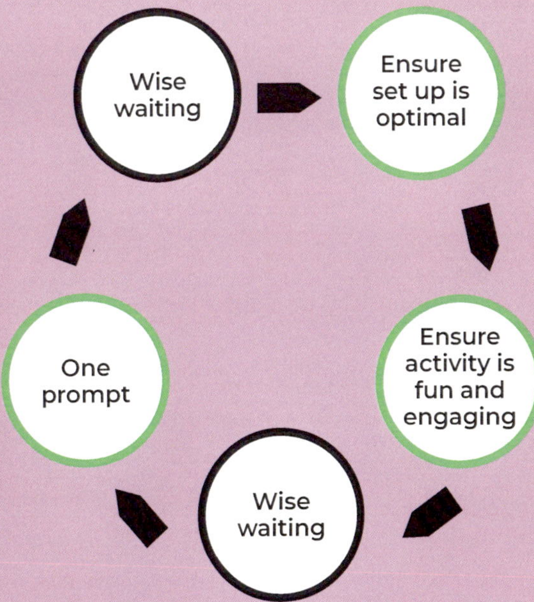

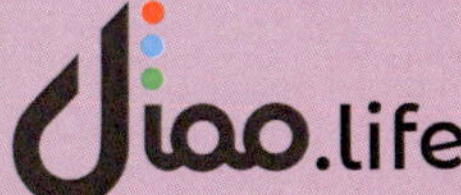

The Assessment Tool

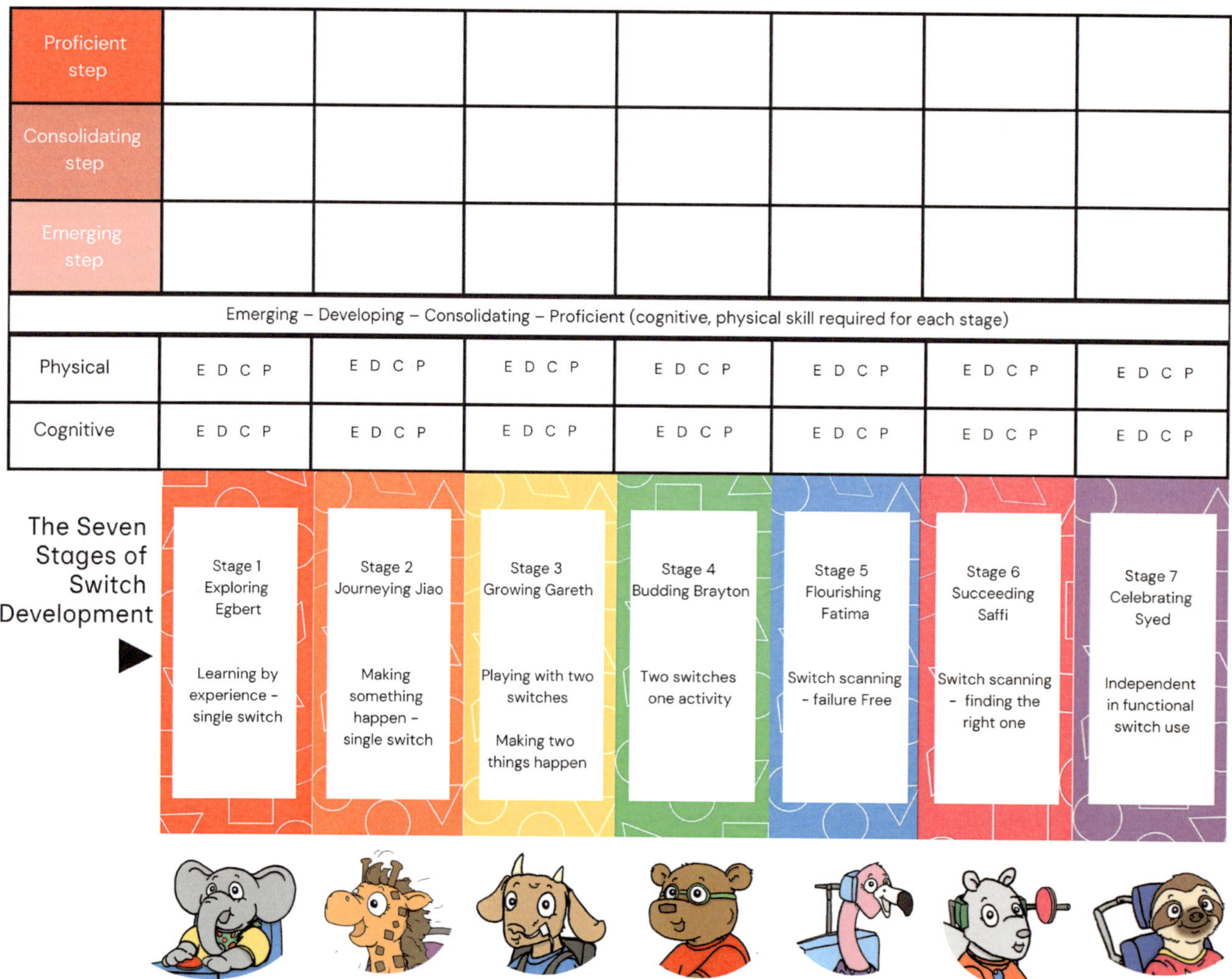

Proficient step							
Consolidating step							
Emerging step							
Emerging – Developing – Consolidating – Proficient (cognitive, physical skill required for each stage)							
Physical	E D C P	E D C P	E D C P	E D C P	E D C P	E D C P	E D C P
Cognitive	E D C P	E D C P	E D C P	E D C P	E D C P	E D C P	E D C P
The Seven Stages of Switch Development ▶	Stage 1 Exploring Egbert Learning by experience - single switch	Stage 2 Journeying Jiao Making something happen - single switch	Stage 3 Growing Gareth Playing with two switches Making two things happen	Stage 4 Budding Brayton Two switches one activity	Stage 5 Flourishing Fatima Switch scanning - failure Free	Stage 6 Succeeding Saffi Switch scanning - finding the right one	Stage 7 Celebrating Syed Independent in functional switch use

Print version available at diao.life

How to use the assessment tool

- The stages of switch development are not mutually exclusive, so progress can be made across multiple stages simultaneously
- Once a step is completed, mark it off and add the date
- The assessment tool can be used for goal setting, where helpers can add target dates and change the text/box colour accordingly
- There is a stream for assessing cognitive and physical skill development, divided into four steps for each stage (Emerging, Developing, Consolidating and Proficient)
- Helpers should consider the cognitive and physical skills required for each level
- This additional stream can help identify areas that may require additional support and highlight strengths and weaknesses for targeted interventions

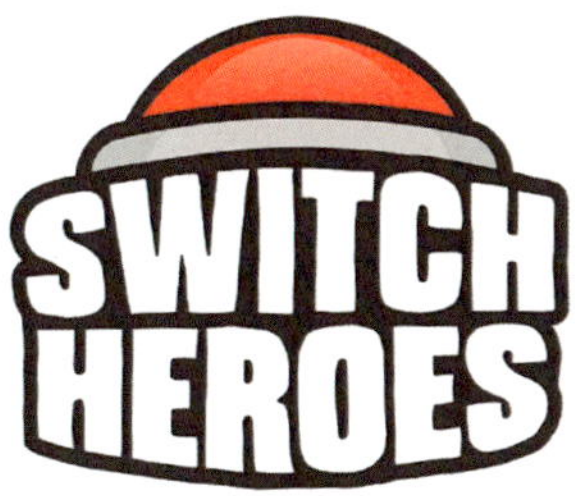

At Jiao Ltd, we are dedicated to empowering individuals through innovative assistive technology solutions.

We provide personalised services and training to help children, families, and professionals navigate the world of assistive tech. For more resources, training options, or to learn how we can support you, visit Jiao.life or get in touch with us directly. We look forward to hearing from you!

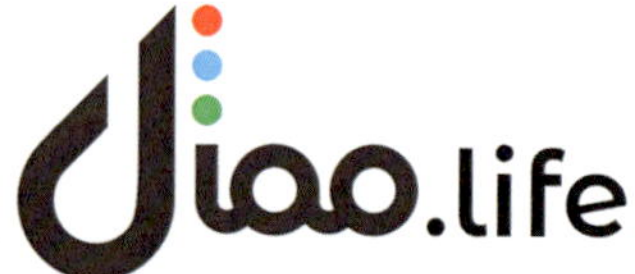

This is to certify that

____

is using two switches

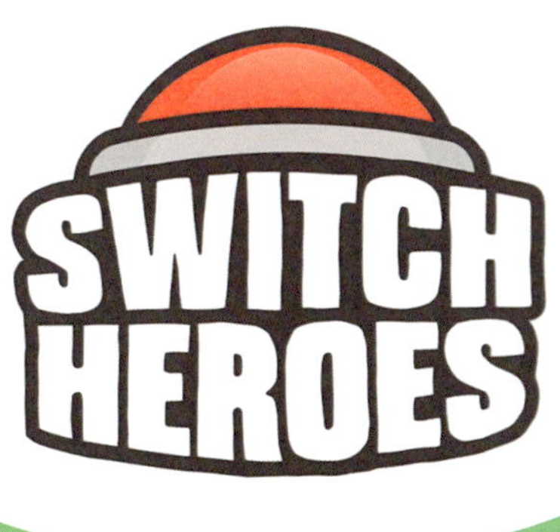

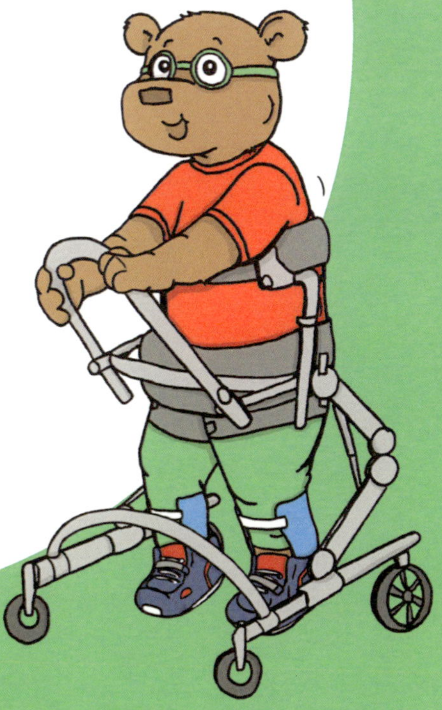

Notes

www.ingramcontent.com/pod-product-compliance
Ingram Content Group UK Ltd.
Pitfield, Milton Keynes, MK11 3LW, UK
UKRC032027290726
14090UKWH00008B/481

* 9 7 8 1 8 0 3 2 9 9 7 6 1 *